CAMERON THANE

FASTING GUIDE

The Ultimate Guide to Intermittent Fasting for Beginners, Discover and Learn All The Information About This Feast and Famine Diet

Descrierea CIP a Bibliotecii Naționale a României
CAMERON THANE
    FASTING GUIDE. The Ultimate Guide to Intermittent Fasting for Beginners, Discover and Learn All The Information About This Feast and Famine Diet / Cameron Thane. – Bucharest: Editura My Ebook, 2020
    ISBN

CAMERON THANE

FASTING GUIDE

The Ultimate Guide to Intermittent Fasting for Beginners, Discover and Learn All The Information About This Feast and Famine Diet

My Ebook Publishing House
Bucharest, 2020

TABLE OF CONTENTS

INTRODUCTION

It's almost impossible to hide from the news and discussion about the obesity epidemic that's taking both lives and shattering the quality of life world wide. It's in the papers, on television and being blogged about on the internet almost endlessly.

If that's not enough, unless you're blind it's hard to walk the streets of any big city or small town and not see the end product of this epidemic first hand.

The hard brutal truth is that people are getting fatter and fatter and this is a real health crisis that only a fool could ignore.

There's plenty of reasons for this here are just the most blindingly apparent...

Many People Eat Way too Much Way too Often.

It's a hard truth that can't be escaped. The human body wasn't designed by nature to eat as much and as often as most people do. This packs on the flabby pounds as our bodies, which are machines that were designed for survival in not so great circumstances are pampered and overfed in a cushy and soft environment. Remove a bit of hunger from our lives and we will pack on fat and pack it on at lightning speed.

A Widespread Avoidance of Exercise.

After overeating the next huge issue is under exercising. Having less physical jobs as well as social lives that revolve around the digital rather than the physical once again takes our bodies away from what they were designed for: running, lifting, hunting and playing. The less muscle we carry the lower our metabolism which means even more fat is packed on. Do you see a pattern developing?

Lack of Quality Sleep.

The first two obesity builders contribute to the third. Poor diet and lack of exercise offer the fast track to broken sleep patterns which have been shown in more studies than can be counted to also wreck metabolism and pack on fat. Sleepless nights tossing and turning quickly equal an ugly spare tire of flab around the waist.

Medicine and Drugs

Coming along with our increasingly over medicated society are the side effects of all these medications, which commonly include weight gain and lethargy. Cultures who approach health more naturally and holistically have largely avoided this issue and have been also able to avoid the obesity related health concerns that come along with it. Our societies for the most part haven't figured this out yet.

These are just some of the many reasons the obesity plague is spreading in such a quick and deadly manner. There's plenty more, trust me.

The question stands - what can we do about it? How can we turn the tide against obesity?

The answer is, of course, diet and exercise. There's plenty of diverse ideas about both, some good and a few bad.

This guide offers what I feel may be the perfect solution to a vast majority of people's struggle with putting on fat. It's fairly simple and packed with power, inline with both nature and common sense. Most importantly it works and works almost like magic.

It's called the Feast and Famine Diet and it can change your life for the better. After reading this you will be armed with all you need to know about Feast and Famine to make it work and get the lean and healthy body of your dreams.

Get ready this is going to be a blast!

CHAPTER 1

WHAT IS THE FEAST AND FAMINE DIET?

The Feast and Famine Diet may be new in name, but in practice has been with us for quite some time. It's the latest tweak on an area of diet programs and ideas less catchingly referred to as Intermittent Fasting.

Intermittent Fasting is the rage in health, fitness and weight loss circles with it's ideas making it to publication and wide practice. It's popular because it works!

Here's the important guiding principles of Feast and Famine, what gives the diet its power. Try not to stray too far from this foundation if you expect to reap the full rewards of Feast and Famine...

Choose Your Fasting Schedule

There's two approaches generally. The first is alternating Feast days with Famine days, which is personally the method I have seen produce the best weight loss results. The second variant, and this is what you will see in intermittent fasting diets like the 5:2 Diet is to eat normally five days and fast two. Our Guide's information works well with both methods, although once again I prefer the first for best long term results as well as ease of use and likelihood of being able to stick with Feast and Famine.

Feasting Guidelines

There's not many. I suggest broadly not eating anything that's junk food or packed with empty calories especially if you are looking to burn off a lot of weight. This will also safeguard your overall health, which is important isn't it? Make sure you get in your fruit and vegetables, but don't be afraid to indulge without binge eating. The fact you have more food freedom at least half the time will make your Famine days much easier to manage psychology.

And succeeding on any diet, Feast and Famine included, is 90% a mental game. In this mental dieting game no diet stacks the deck more in your favor than Feast and Famine.

Famine Guidelines

For those needing to drop serious pounds, 500 calories a day on Famine days is a good starting point. This can be adjusted as needed once your weight loss goals are met. Most Feast and Famine enthusiasts like to stay around this area to continue to both reap the health benefits of fasting and to also be able to maintain their Feasting freedom on their Feast days.

* Stay Hydrated. Fasting expert or if you have never fasted in any form before alike, I cannot stress enough the importance of staying hydrated. When your body detoxes on your Famine days and starts to move out some of the junk you have built up, it will go much smoother if you are drinking a proper amount of water. Ignore this advice and you may just experience some stomach pains, along with the lethargy and weakness that always comes with dehydration regardless of your diet plan.

One of the greatest strengths of intermittent fasting and the Feast and Famine Diet is its simplicity. No diet logs, carbohydrate manipulation schemes and other complications. It works much more dramatically than diets that you need flow charts to follow too. If you can't stick to Feast and Famine it has nothing to do with being confused, but with a lack of will power, self discipline and most of all desire. I think you have those covered, don't you?

CHAPTER 2

THE BEGINNING OF THE FEAST & FAMINE DIET

Every good idea got its start somewhere. The every other day Feast and Famine Diet has had its way paved for it by earlier intermittent fasting protocols, some a big influence and others not so much, but who still deserve credit for being forward thinkers.

Let's take a look at the history of diets that have come before Feast and Famine and see what we can learn from them. Knowledge is power after all. We have already seen in the mirror and felt in our bodies - that Feast and Famine works big time, we have these pace setters to thank for their experiments and innovations!

First The Warrior.

Make no mistake, Ori Hofmekler is certainly a unique guy. Artist, writer and ex-special forces soldier who ran a short lived fitness magazine that was published by a famous Men's magazine company.

During his time as editor in chief he was exposed to the often conflicting ideas of a who's who of dieting gurus of the time, which landed him an obsession with getting to the truth about fat loss.

A few years later came the Warrior Diet book which promotes a 16 hour daily fast followed by a 8 hour eating period. Overall consensus was that it worked, but most people feel the Warrior Diet is difficult to maintain, much more so than every other day fasting ala Feast and Famine. Either way Ori definitely get's credit for the modern birth of intermittent fasting and has served as a great influence on most everyone's ideas who are working with these methods.

Eat Stop Eat.

Eat Stop Eat has been an intermittent fasting dieting method promoted most recently by Brad Pillon. Brad pushes the idea of one or two, zero calorie days a week, the rest of the days eating normally. Once again it's effective and close to what we suggest, but our experience has shown going down to 500 calories every other day is much more effective and manageable than a few days of no calories at all. Not many seem to be able to stick with Eat Stop Eat for long in our experience.

The 5:2 Diet.

This is the diet plan most closely related to Feast and Famine and also closest to us on the time line. It's wildly popular in Europe and is gaining ground in places like Hollywood in the USA.

Five days of normal eating followed by two days of reduced calories. Very powerful and all our ideas here work well with the 5:2 Diet. Our opinion holds every other day Feast and Famine is a better fat burner without added psychological tolls. Follow this Guide's advice and I think you will agree!

That's the recent history of intermittent fasting leading us to where we are today. Feast and Famine is the present and I have no doubt it will proudly stand the test of time. It torches fat, is easy to follow, requires really no added expenses in its purest form and promotes over all vibrant health. What's there not to love about Feast and Famine? It's perfect for the health enthusiast who wants to get lean and look great.

CHAPTER 3

THE BENEFITS OF THE FEAST & FAMINE DIET

The Feast and Famine Diet brings a load of benefits some more obvious than others. Are you ready to take a look? I think you'll find them really exciting. If radically reducing fat while also basking in these health benefits doesn't interest someone looking to transform their body for the better I'm not sure what will!

Quickly Cut Body Fat Safely

This is why most people will explore the Feast and Famine approach to diet. You can expect to see the fat melt off as long as you take your Famine days seriously. Eat too much on those days and you are obviously missing the point. We know this works, we've seen it and now even better news - science backs it up!

Recent University of Illinois research has shown in those following alternate day reduced calorie plans (inline with our Guide's recommendations) **lost significantly more fat** than those eating normally and following the same exercise protocols. It's a plus to be on the right side of science when, sadly, they most often trail far behind the true health and diet vanguard!

Easy To Follow And Manage

The next ground breaking benefit of Feast and Famine is how easy it is to follow and manage. I've touched on this already, but it truly bears repeating. Anyone who has counted carbs on a ketogenic diet like Atkins or the many others I'm sure will quickly agree! Once you figure out in your head what your 500 or 600 calories on famine days looks like you are set. No calculators or complications, period.

Enhanced Mental Function

Yes, we suspected it, but science has backed us up again. Reduced weekly calories (which is what you get with the Feast and Famine Diet) leads to increased focus, better memory and other enhanced cognitive function according to Mark Mattson's research for the Lancet. These effects may even carry over into the fight against Alzheimer's disease and other similar huge health concerns which Mattson is exploring further.

Improve Insulin Levels

One of the reasons why many people pack on and find it so hard to lose body fat is their out of whack insulin levels. The Feast and Famine approach optimizes insulin levels for healthy fat loss, which just adds to the amount of fat already being cut from the calorie reduction and heightened metabolism we've already touched on.

Frees Up Time On Famine Days

One of the surprise benefits of this approach is the new found time you find available on Famine days. Small meals and no constant snacking or grazing frees up a shocking amount of time and energy that can be used positively elsewhere. I've found, and others have confirmed this, that some of our most creative and productive days turn out again and again to be famine days! Far from not having energy you end up filled with it!

The Feast and Famine Diet approach is packed with benefits, physical, mental and even social. It's hard to even think of anything, but a small drawback or two and then only for those who are lacking in the desire to "get lean" department. This is truly a method that changes lives for the best.

CHAPTER 4

GETTING YOURSELF READY TO BEGIN

Any diet requires a bit of preparation at first, Feast and Famine is certainly not an exception. I will say it requires much less preparation by the nature of Feast and Famine than any other diet I can think of and you won't have to jump many hurdles, do any real expensive shopping or experience any of the other more traditional diet head aches.

Here's some tips to get yourself ready to get the most out our plan...

Read And Understand This Guide

It's pretty short so why not even read it twice. I've done my best to keep it fluff free and all the information and tips will make your journey at intermittent fasting Feast and Famine style much, much easier. If you like to read check out some of the books in our history chapter and you may find some other ideas you'd like to incorporate after you've done straight Feast and Famine for a bit.

If Possible At First Food Shop More Often

Here's a trick I used in the beginning days of my intermittent fasting experiments and I've suggested to many of my friends and clients who have given it high praise too. Only keep enough food on hand for the days needs. On Feasting days you will have the pleasure of picking out some new treat to indulge in and on Famine days you won't be as tempted to cheat than you would be if the refrigerator is packed with snacks. Now if you live rurally, or have a large family this may be less practical, but if you can do it I guarantee it will give you a big advantage over those who ignore this tip.

If You Skip A Day Just Get Right Back On Schedule

This diet is about freedom and abundance not restriction. If you have a family event, a date or even a slight slip up on a Famine day just get right back in action the next day and reduce your calories. No master dietary equations are fouled or other nonsense. Now don't make a habit of this or you may end up seeing less than optimal results, but once in a while is perfectly fine. This automatic leeway is built into the Feast and Famine program making it not a diet you can "fail" at if you stumble while getting into the groove, or any other time really!

Throw Out Your Past Diet Experiences

Feast and Famine requires a whole new view of dieting, so in all likelihood your past dieting experiences positive and especially negative don't offer a whole lot of relevance. I'd suggest you file them away and don't let them influence what you are doing here and now. This attitude, not only in dieting and fitness, but also in other areas of life can break chains and open up doors. See what you think.

Are you feeling more ready to begin? You should be because there's a bright, fit and happy new you waiting at the end of the Feast and Famine road. And it's a road not particularly long in most cases or even exceedingly difficult. You've taken the first step by reading this Guide, don't turn back now!

CHAPTER 5

COMMON BEGINNER MISTAKES

Now just because the Feast and Famine Diet is easy to understand and simple to apply to your lifestyle doesn't mean it's easy for all to practice or it's impossible to make mistakes. In fact some mistakes with intermittent fasting are fairly common among beginners, let's go over them and see if you can't avoid these pitfalls before you make them rather than after. A few of these I even learned the hard way!

Pigging Out on Too Much on Junk Food

Let's be serious for a second on the subject of getting lean and healthy. While we are allowed and encouraged to eat loosely and enjoyably on Feast days this doesn't mean we have a license to eat completely like a glutton. So if you are not losing weight the way you'd like to be and are eating endless chips, ice cream and candy on your Feast days tighten up your diet and eat healthier.

You should be striving to optimize your health anyway shouldn't you?

Being Scared to Death of Hunger

No one has ever starved to death eating 500 calories or less every other day. Nor have they damaged their body in any way. So if you are experiencing great stress and discomfort over being hungry every other day, it's time to gain more control over your mind. This is done by developing your will power doing things like following this diet even when you would rather not be, focusing on your desired end result. Be tough and be rewarded.

Eating Too Much On Famine Days

Let's not play games, 500 calories or less means 500 calories or less. If you are eating clean on your Feast days and still not losing weight it likely means you are eating too much on Famine days. Cut down what you are eating and if you must check the calorie counts to make sure you are at 500 calories or under.

Reducing Your Level of Activity

It's tempting for some to slow down their activities on Famine days. Don't fall into this. In fact with a little Feast and Famine experience under your belt you will realize Famine days actually free up more energy and you should strive to be even more active. Doing more is almost always better than doing nothing as long as you can do it safely.

Putting Yourself Unnecessarily Around People Who Don't Respect Your Diet Efforts.

Apart from close friends and family who it would be difficult to avoid, it's a downer to be around people who try to talk negatively about or discourage you from meeting your Feast and Famine goals. Again dieting is 90% mental so don't let other people mess with your mental game. It's annoying, defeatist and unnecessary!

These common beginner mistakes are all easy to avoid and if you stumble it's ok just keep going. The Feast and Famine Diet has been designed to be both effective, open and user friendly. A little bit of self-reflection and you are quickly back on course and seizing the body and life of your dreams!

CHAPTER 6

A SAMPLE FEAST DAY

The Feast and Famine Feast Day! Now comes the fun part, my friends! Let's dig deep into a sample Feast day while we are following the Feast and Famine Diet.

This is taken from my own lifestyle and from a period of time when I was consistently losing weight as fast as I ever had every week without fail. My metabolism has never been superhuman either, so rest assured if this has worked for me it's very, very likely to work for you as well (with portion sizes adjusted if you are female, of course.)

Read on and enjoy. I hope it gets you filled with enthusiasm! You will notice I'm not including calories, because who counts calories on a Feast day?! I sure don't and you shouldn't either.

Breakfast

Breakfast is regarded by many nutrition experts as being the most important meal of the day. It's also a meal I've neglected most of my life due to the perils of enjoying sleeping in. Intermittent fasting has cleared that up - after a 500 calorie day I can't wait to really eat a substantial breakfast! I must say I feel much more ready for action after a full force breakfast.

4 Eggs Scrambled. I choose to go with whole eggs for hormonal optimization's sake, but often mix up the ways the eggs are prepared.

Fresh Tomato, Onion and Jalapeno Salsa. Extra hot and used as a condiment on top of my eggs.

4 pieces of Turkey Bacon. I will eat other styles of bacon when turkey bacon isn't available.

4oz of Steak Sauteed in Frying Pan. I only add this when I really want to indulge or if I feel like I need the extra protein for muscle building purposes.

8oz Milk. Whole milk is also great for guys looking to naturally boost their hormonal advantage,

Snack

A few hand fulls of Organic Almonds

Small Spinach Salad. I don't use dressing beyond olive oil and garlic and sometimes toss in some tomatoes, onion and cucumber depending what's on hand.

Lunch

Medium Baked Potato. I dress the potato with a bit of butter and garlic.

Two 6oz Grilled Chicken Breasts. Sometimes plain or sometimes with salsa on top if I have extra from breakfast.

Small Side of Mixed Vegetables. Snack More Almonds!

Dinner

10oz Grilled Lean Steak. Plain beyond salt and pepper.

Small side salad or spinach salad. Side Portion of White or Brown Rice.

As much **Green Tea** as I'd like to drink sweetened with pure stevia.

Occasionally a desert of organic sorbet, a small addiction of mine!

Snack

My after dinner snack is pretty wide open within reason. If I eat chips I make sure to not go overboard.

Vanilla Whey Protein shake made with half whole milk and half almond milk. I drink this right before bed.

This is just a sample Feast and Famine Feast day, but it should give you a great idea of what's possible when we eat smartly and abundantly. The real eye opener is when you eat like this half the time and still see the fat melting away. That's when you will become a full force Feast and Famine true believer!

CHAPTER 7

A SAMPLE FAMINE DAY

Now after seeing a sample Feast and Famine Feast day it's time for a sample of the flip side - the all important Famine day where we will fast eating vastly reduced calories activating our metabolism, our "skinny gene" and setting ourselves up for both body transformation and all the other health benefits we have already discussed. This is again, from my own personal experience and the daily calorie total is focused on the magic number of 500 calories. I think you will find this a very manageable day that will hardly leave you suffering.

Pre-Breakfast

16oz Spring Water immediately upon wakening.

A cup of Fresh Coffee, no milk or cream sweetened with stevia. 0 calories.

Breakfast

A second cup of Fresh Coffee, no milk or cream sweetened with stevia. 0 calories.

8oz Spring Water.

Now this doesn't seem like much of a breakfast, but I prefer to sleep in a bit and save my calories for lunch and dinner. This is my own personal choice and you may choose to distribute your calories differently if you are more of a morning person!

Snack

8oz Green Tea sweetened with stevia. 0 calories.

12oz Spring water. Lunch

Finally time to get in some food, paying special intention NOT to over do it. This is the meal when many feel most tempted, since while eating a small dinner you know a large breakfast is coming up relatively quickly. Don't give in!

Two medium hard boiled eggs. Once again I like to make sure I eat whole eggs every day to maximize my hormonal optimization plan. You have the option of egg whites, egg beaters and so on. 175 Calories.

Two slices Whole Wheat Toast. Sometimes I eat the eggs on the toast and sometimes as a side depending on mood. 115 Calories.

A cup of Fresh Coffee, no milk or cream sweetened with stevia. 0 calories.

8oz spring water.

Total Lunch calories: 290 give or take.

Snack

8oz Green Tea sweetened with stevia. 0 calories. Yes, I do love caffeine on Famine day in case you were wondering. It serves to boost energy, raise metabolism and even acts as a mild appetite suppressant.

12oz Spring water. Dinner

Half a cup (after cooked) Spaghetti with a small amount of low fat / low calorie butter, salt, pepper and garlic. 150 calories.

One slice whole wheat toast. 55 calories.

12oz Spring Water.

Total calorie intake for the day roughly 495 calories. This puts right where we are hoping to be on a Famine day. I repeat these meals often since they are pretty much decision free and simple to prepare. They can also easily be ordered in all but the most incompetent of restaurants!

One last bit of advice - take a half hour on Sunday and figure out your five hundred calorie and below meals for the week rather than just trying to wing it and guess how many calories you are eating on Famine days on the fly.

This will end up equating in much more weight loss over the long term and also save you a few head aches and a bit of possible confusion too. When in doubt repeat meals! Don't worry about getting bored a Feast day is less than 24 hours away!

CHAPTER 8

SHOPPING GUIDELINES

Now that we hopefully have agreed that the Feast and Famine Diet is more than do-able after looking at a sample Feast day and a sample Famine day I thought I'd share with you a few more intermittent fasting insider's secrets.

The fine art of shopping while following Feast and Famine. Although all of us develop our style of eating while on the diet which best suits our individual needs I've found having an experience veteran's shopping list can provide some helpful guidelines. So are you ready to go shopping Feast and Famine style? Let's do it!

Here's what we are packing our shopping cart with...

Non-hormonal Chicken Breasts. I'm a bit of a chicken addict and don't think I could live without it. I eat chicken at least once a day on Feast days, sometimes twice. I think of chicken as a sort of "neutral" protein that can be prepared in so many ways its wise to fall in love with.

Make sure the fat is trimmed off!

Non-hormonal Grass Fed Lean Beef. Another Feast day favorite, especially when I'm hitting it more heavily in the gym. When you are looking to put on muscle while cutting fat on Feast and Famine aim for around 1 gram of protein for every pound you weigh.

Eggs. As you've seen eggs are on the meal agenda often for both Feast and Famine days. Don't skip them, unless you are one of the few who can't stomach the thought of them!

A variety of Pasta. Organic Spinach

Organic Leaf Lettuce. I should add organic produce is not a must, but I try to stick with it when I can.

Tomatoes.

Onions.

Miso soup. Miso soup is great for a change of pace on Famine days and has been shown in research to have all sorts of regenerative and health boosting qualities. Plus it tastes great too!

Green Tea. Essential. Green Tea is great for a extra fat burning boost, is inexpensive and calorie free.

Coffee. Spring Water.

Whey Protein. I've tried to avoid any supplement recommendations as the Feast and Famine Diet works great without them, but a good protein shake is the one exception. Keep your protein levels high and you will have no worries at all about losing muscle while cutting body fat.

Stevia. A all natural and calorie free sweetener which will make you forget sugar ever even existed. A true gift from above.

Almonds. A go to snack.

Now a look at this list reveals that avoiding overly processed and junk food isn't a bad idea and you can still really Feast without it. That way if you go a bit crazy at a friend's or eating out occasionally your body won't even notice it. Buying too many terrible food choices probably sends the wrong message to your subconscious and may set up many for binge eating and failure. Some intermittent fasting experts disagree, but this is what my own personal experience has revealed. After you move beyond the beginner stage feel free to experiment!

CHAPTER 9

INCORPORATING THE FEAST & FAMINE DIET
INTO YOUR LIFESTYLE LONGTERM

The only way to really lose weight and keep it off is to make the mental switch from thinking in terms of short term dieting to the more dynamic perspective of making lasting healthy lifestyle choices.

Feast and Famine is the perfect tool to help you make that change. In fact after studying and experimenting with every major diet of the last decade, I can honestly say none in my opinion are better suited for a long term lifestyle choice than intermittent fasting and Feast and Famine. It's easy to manage, inexpensive to follow, relatively pleasant and enjoyable and very, very powerful. This covers nearly every category of a dream long term eating plan check list I can think of!

Here's some tips in incorporating Feast and Famine into your lifestyle long term...

Celebrate Your Successes With Feast And Famine.

Thinking positive and choosing to focus on the positive changes you have made while intermittent fasting will go a long way in solidifying it as a part of your lasting lifestyle. Try your best to not dwell on any poor weeks or bumps in the road you may experience. This will pay off huge dividends both in weight loss and in life. Again 90% of the game is mental, let's not forget.

Recruit Those Closest To You To Lend A Hand

Making your significant other close friends and family aware of how Feast and Famine works and letting them know you could use their help encouraging you to be disciplined on Famine days will help this healthy lifestyle really cement itself in place. Some may even choose to take up the Feast and Famine flag themselves when they see how great you look and feel. That's when you know you are really onto something!

Take Off A Week Off Every Few Months

Everyone needs a vacation occasionally. This will prevent burn out and give yourself a great pat on the back after months of discipline. If you can time your vacation from Feast and Famine with a real vacation from work or school even better! I've found a week off really helps recharge enthusiasm's batteries and allows me to plunge back into the Feast and Famine lifestyle full force.

Keep Expanding Your Knowledge Of Intermittent Fasting

A final way to make sure you stick with Feast and Famine as a lifestyle choice is to keep your brain engaged in learning new knowledge about intermittent fasting in all its forms. Join some forums, follow the news and the blogs and if you go to a gym make friends with others living this way of life. This will continually confirm what you are doing is both healthy and a good choice. It's always a good idea to have as big a support circle as possible.

Even if you take up Feast and Famine to lose some weight quickly planning to go back to your old ways of eating, let me

43

warn you, you may very well end up hooked and sticking around for the duration. The good news is your body will be much healthier and look much better for your efforts. Breaking from the norm into a lifestyle that gets the most out of body and mind is a benefit that's priceless. Embrace it!

CONCLUSION

TIPS TO BEGIN YOUR DIET JOURNEY TODAY

Thanks for taking the time to read our Guide and I truly hope you have found it helpful and eye opening. I have no doubt if you throw your focus into the Feast and Famine Diet you will achieve your weight loss goals and much more.

That said when do you plan to start? If you just hesitated you may be experiencing the greatest foe of achieving the body of your dreams of them all - the evil called procrastination. Before I leave let me share with you some tips that can help you slay that beast and begin your own transformation story today!

Just Do It

The Feast and Famine Diet requires no special food, no supplements and no information, really, beyond this Guide to work and work well. So what are you waiting for? Start Feast and Famine right NOW. The only thing stopping you is your own inertia. Banish any thoughts of tomorrow or next week. Once again make a decision and start NOW.

Expose Your Excuses

Do you have reoccurring excuses why you can't start intermittent fasting today? Say these excuses out loud so you can hear how ridiculously self defeating they are. If you are still in doubt write them down and burn them as you free yourself from limiting beliefs.

Look At Yourself Naked In The Mirror.

If you are fat the mirror and a lack of clothes won't lie. Remind yourself your body won't change into something more pleasing until you first make a decision to change it and then second move forward with action in support of that decision. That action is to wisely adopt the Feast and Famine Diet. If not you will likely look the same, if not worse, than you did in the mirror in the days, weeks, months and years to come. This may sound harsh, but a harsh truth is much better than a pleasant falsehood.

Quit Time Wasters.

Do you need so much social media, television or playing video games when your body isn't where you desire it to be? Are you putting the easy and distracting before the vital and important? If so why? Break the trance, quit the time wasters and build the new you NOW!

Write Your Goals Down As Clearly And Detailed As Possible.

There's a certain magic about the written word, especially when it comes to setting and achieving goals. This magic is even more pronounced when the written words are your own. Write down your goals big and small, read them and embrace Feast and Famine as a means to carry you in the direction you need to be headed. There isn't a success coach or sports psychologist alive who would argue against that advice! You shouldn't either.

Are you psyched about moving forward with Feast and Famine? I knew you would be. This could be a day you look back on decades from now and say "that's where I committed to serious life enhancing change!" The things offered by this lifestyle are just that serious. I'd love to hear your success story so please stay strong and in touch!

Printed by Libri Plureos GmbH in Hamburg,
Germany

9 786069 836446